I WANT TO GET FIT

Katy Bircher & Katie Goodwin

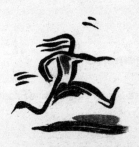

SUMMERSDALE

Summersdale Publishers Ltd
46 West Street
Chichester
West Sussex
PO19 1RP
United Kingdom

www.summersdale.com

Printed and bound in Great Britain by Cox & Wyman.

ISBN 1 84024 063 6

Acknowledgements

Our thanks go to Sarah Hill , Claire Frost, George Peck and Michelle Cross.

Illustrations by Robert Bircher.

Contents

Introduction

If you're reading this then you are either a) one of our
friends and you've been given a free copy in the hope
that your comments will boost our egos, or b) someone
who has decided that you can no longer ignore the
approach or manifestation of the changes of an ageing
body.

It is Sod's law that as you grow older, while your life
and career may begin to take shape and your self-
confidence increases, your body starts to fall apart.
Bits appear that were never there in childhood, or even
in those dodgy teenage years. You are convinced that
that dimple in your backside was smaller yesterday;
you wonder how on earth that cellulite could have been
allowed to creep up on you and attach itself to the
back of your legs. And when was it that running for a
bus became such hard work? How can, 'Let's all go to
the park and play football this afternoon' be so
completely uninspiring? The changes come upon you
secretly, mischievously, and before you know it you

have become UNFIT, lethargic, flabby, and you really have no idea what additional horrors you'll discover if you catch sight of yourself in that full-length mirror tomorrow.

If you recognise any of these feelings then it's time to act. If you recognise them from five years ago but have managed so far to ignore them, then seize the day. You are completely normal. Absolutely everyone goes through this, but only a few manage really to take control and begin a fitness programme that lasts. Try to make sure you become one of them – we promise it will be worth it.

Healthy Body, Healthy Mind

People who have got themselves fit will tell you that, 'I just feel so much better...' often with a slightly bemused look in their eyes. Can physical fitness make you feel like a more complete person? Are you really more likely to feel better about yourself, because you do four classes a week at your local gym? Neither of us are scientists with surveys and statistics at our fingertips but the answer from our own experience has to be an emphatic 'YES'.

In the year 4BC Plato argued that his students should be sent 'to the master of gymnastics in order that their bodies may better minister to the virtuous mind.' Similarly, in the year 2BC, Galen asserted that 'exercise is recommended which contributes to the health of the body and to the harmonious functioning of the parts and to the strength of the soul.' In modern times, there have been over a hundred separate studies, which have statistically established the correlation between a happy and satisfactory state of mind and good physical health. Put simply, if you feel good physically then you're more likely to feel both mentally and emotionally healthier.

Why does fitness affect your state of mind?

• *Exercise converts adrenaline into energy*

It is known that when we are under stress – perhaps due to personal problems, general work pressures, deadlines, an annoying boss – our brain signals for the production of *catecholamines*, or adrenaline. Adrenaline causes a heightened stimulation, usually increasing the sense of anxiety, certainly provoking higher blood pressure and an increased heart rate. During regular exercise this adrenaline can be converted into energy; it is used as a fuel and burned up along the way. Therefore regular exercise can be said to release the pressure valve, allowing some of our tension out in a healthy and controlled way.

• *Exercise causes the brain to secrete endorphins*

Exercise also provokes a natural 'high' caused by the brain's secretion of *endorphins* – morphine-like chemicals that help combat pain and stress. It is this 'buzz' that many fitness fanatics become addicted to, but as long as your reaction to it does not become obsessive, endorphins give you a healthy sense of wellbeing.

- ### *Exercise is our body's traditional way of coping during difficult times*

  Our physicality is a vital part of our experience as humans and 70% of our body is given over to the purpose of movement. Before the onset of modern civilisation we were hunter-gatherers, needing physical endurance and strength to find food and to survive. Perhaps the recognition of a desire to get fit even today is a response to a primitive need for survival. This might explain why the desire often kicks in in times of crisis or despair, as if our DNA is telling us that exercise is a way of coping on a very basic level – simply of surviving through a difficult time.

- ### *Exercise promotes self-confidence.*

  Perhaps our perception of quality of life is closely linked with the knowledge that we are making the best of our available hereditary characteristics. Certainly there is something deeply satisfying about realising our potential, doing our best, making the most of what we have. This in turn increases our feelings of self-worth and self-confidence because we feel good about ourselves.

- ### *Exercise makes you feel alive*

  The centres of the brain that manage and co-ordinate our muscular actions are anatomically very close to the centres that manage feeling and thinking. The possibility that one brain centre could positively affect another is large, and a tingling sense of being alive might very well be our feeling brain centre's response to the muscular brain centre's activity.

Such explanations for the feel-good factor of exercise are useful. It is good to understand what may be happening in your brain as you get fit and, scientifically, to see the very possible connection between a healthy body and a healthy mind.

However, much of this remains unknown to the average gym-goer, and we have found that, far more persuasive and conclusive than any study or survey, is the obvious positive change in the way we feel on a basic day to day level. Again we return to the slightly bemused 'I just feel so much better' assertion. Most importantly, we both feel the pride of having really taken control of this aspect of our lives; it has become something that is ours, done for ourselves and done in the way that we wanted to. When you are trying, for whatever reason, to assert your own identity, to establish a sense of self-worth and self-confidence – getting fit helps enormously.

Warning

We would like to conclude this section with a couple of warnings against obsessive fitness. Neither of us are obsessive about fitness – any sort of obsession only serves to make you miserable – but the temptation in today's society is to seek quick remedies and packaged answers to all kinds of problems.

Many people fall into the trap of trying to do too much too quickly – eight classes a week, no food for three days, no sweets or treats at all. It's easy to be drawn to this way of thinking, particularly at the beginning of a fitness programme when you've reached desperation and want change FAST, but it doesn't work. It is unsustainable and you will give up before any real benefit has been established. Go slowly and surely. Remember the hare and the tortoise.

The Physical Benefits of Exercise

As well as the all round psychological benefits of fitness, there is, of course, the whole subject of our health. The realisation that good health – which many of us have been happy to take for granted – is not guaranteed to continue is perhaps beginning to dawn. Reminders that we must be more considerate towards our bodies on matters of exercise and nutrition become increasingly pressing. Just some of the benefits inherent in exercise include the fact that it:

- Helps fight arterial disease
- Lowers blood pressure
- Improves circulation
- Promotes weight loss

Fitness & Evolution

Throughout our evolution, humans have had to depend on their muscular ability for survival, making physical fitness a necessity, but we have now arrived at a time where we are rarely required to call on this natural potential. Travel on foot has become a rare and rather quaint idea – a walk in the park is either a special treat or a chore endured for the sake of the dog. The nightmare of running for a bus is, of course, exactly what it says – running a short distance in order to sit and be carried the rest of the journey, not running (or even walking) the entire journey as our ancestors would have done.

Pushing the trolley round the supermarket once in a while is hardly the same as giving chase to a mammoth. Similarly, tapping a few keys on the computer and printing out multiple copies is not comparable with scratching away for hours on end with your quill and ink – or even biro. So it is not surprising to learn that many of our modern day ills are attributable to the use of artificial energy sources rather than our own muscles. However, the state of our muscles is only a small part of physical well being, the main concern being cardiovascular fitness i.e. that concerning the heart and blood.

Heart Disease

Heart disease is one of the biggest causes of premature death and, apart from heredity, the two factors that affect the heart and the blood are:

• Physical activity
• Nutrition

In other words, we can take steps towards protecting ourselves.

Cardiovascular Fitness

The immediate source of energy for muscular activity is *Adenosine Triphosphate* or ATP, of which small amounts are found in resting muscles – enough to support a very limited amount of exercise. Beyond this, the body needs to resynthesise ATP, a process that requires oxygen for the release of energy in the breakdown of carbohydrates and fats stored in the body. Carbohydrate is transported by the blood in the form of glucose (blood sugar) and is either used immediately for energy or converted into glycogen for storage. Fats are transported as fatty acids and if not used are stored in layers under the skin.

The more strenuous the exercise, the more oxygen used and carbon dioxide produced. In a healthy person it is generally thought that neither the lungs nor the ventilation muscles put any restriction on activity, so you don't need special exercises to increase their capacity. Most importantly, the heart's ability to pump the blood can be increased, resulting in the availability of more oxygen to working muscles. This chain of events comes from the stamina training or *aerobic exercise* (so called because of the involvement of oxygen in the movement of the muscles).

Fifteen to twenty minutes of fairly vigorous aerobic exercise three times a week is enough to encourage various muscular changes: the muscles increase their capacity for taking in oxygen by producing more *mitochondria* (the sites which produce the ATP which produce energy) and therefore the oxygen is used more efficiently. The changes to the muscles in turn affect the heart, which pumps more blood with every beat, meaning that it has to do less to achieve the same output and can therefore keep going longer.

Heart Rate

The heart rate (pulse) is a good indication of stamina. A fit person has a relatively small rise in heart rate during exercise, which will drop back to normal fairly quickly afterwards, whereas someone who is unfit will find their heart racing during exercise and will find that it takes longer to return to normal.

So it seems to be fairly clear that exercise can be extremely beneficial to our hearts and circulation and for many of us, the idea of burning off fat is a welcome one. It makes sense that if our food intake is much greater than our fuel requirements (i.e. if we eat a lot and don't do much exercise) the excess is stored in fat deposits and some is laid down in the walls of the arteries.

Exercise and Appetite

It is a common concern among those toying with the notion of getting fit, that exercise will only serve to make one hungrier, resulting in the consumption of more food, resulting in a gain in weight, so really let's just not bother at all! This is not a valid argument against getting fit.

Aerobic exercise speeds up the *metabolic rate* (i.e. the rate at which food is converted into energy) not only during exercise, but also for up to 24 hours afterwards. This means that, as an active person, you can be using more calories (or energy) resting in front of the television than your unfit friend – even if he or she is on a diet.

If you need further persuasion, consider the following:

- Exercise raises your blood sugar level and it is a drop in your blood sugar level that causes the feeling of hunger.

- Exercise raises the body temperature: increased body temperature is a natural appetite depressor.

- Regular exercise makes us more aware of how much food our bodies actually require, which prevents unnecessary overeating.

More Benefits of Exercise...

However, these are by no means the only benefits of exercise – the list goes on. As well as helping to fight arterial disease, lowering blood pressure, improving circulation and promoting weight loss, exercise can also:

- Boost your immune system.
- Improve your posture, through the strengthening of muscles to support the spine, preventing or alleviating back pain (one of the most common causes of absence from work).
- Slow or reverse the loss of minerals from bones that may prevent osteoporosis in later life.
- Infinitely increase your self-confidence.

There are so many factors in life, particularly regarding health, that are beyond our control, that it makes sense to invest in our fitness while we can.

Fit For What?

Defining what it actually means to be fit is rather difficult. Reaching an absolute peak of fitness and pushing the body to every one of its limits is unnecessary unless you are planning to take part in the next Olympics or have decided to turn professional and earn millions playing for Arsenal. We would advise you to set your sights a tad lower than this and be a little bit more realistic in your objectives. Obviously, if you've already packed your suitcase for Sydney 2000, this is probably not the book for you.

For us mere mortals, fitness need not be an ultimate, a 'peak', an 'optimum', a 'maximum', or any other scarily serious word. Being fit is about doing an amount of exercise which makes you healthy, gives you more energy, more strength and increased suppleness.

Measuring exact fitness is difficult unless you want to invest in hugely expensive equipment to carry out *VO2 Max tests* or *Bleep tests* – which measure aerobic power and circulatory efficiency. The best scale to work with is a personal one. Simply compare the way you feel on day one of your exercise programme with the way that you feel one month later. You *will* notice a difference. You will know you are getting fitter because things get slowly easier and you start to really enjoy your chosen form of exercise.

Physical Fitness

Physical fitness can be separated into these five categories:

- Aerobic Power
- Strength
- Local Muscle Endurance
- Flexibility
- Body Composition

- **Aerobic Power** is cardiovascular fitness. Aerobic exercises are a type of exercise that work the heart muscle and make it stronger and healthier. During an exercise programme that concentrates on aerobic power, the heart becomes able to pump larger quantities of blood and can therefore process greater amounts of oxygen. The end result is the ability to exercise at increased intensity for longer periods of time – basically, you can do more without getting out of breath and, once you are out of breath, it takes less time to get it back. Your blood vessels become more efficient and they increase in elasticity, size and number – this helps in the battle against heart disease. As the quality of your blood improves, so the red blood cells and haemoglobin – which carry oxygen – become more developed.

- **Strength** is muscle power. Strength is improved by types of exercise which increase the force that a muscle or muscle group can apply. You really need to work with weights to get stronger. A programme of weight training makes your muscles firmer and larger because weight training causes a gradual thickening of the muscle cell walls, an increase in the fluid content of the muscle cells and an increase in the number of blood vessels in the muscle cell.

  Weight training can help you appear thinner as muscles take up less space than fat does. You can lose inches, but you are less likely to lose actual weight because muscle itself is quite heavy. Weight training gives you an increased muscular awareness which helps with general co-ordination and body control, and can greatly improve your posture as you start to become aware of using the correct muscles for even simple things like standing and sitting.

- **Local Muscle Endurance (LME)** is more about toning the muscles by working them over longer periods of time. Whereas *strength* training requires low repetitions against high resistance – i.e. you lift a really heavy weight a small number of times – LME requires higher repetitions against lower resistance – you lift a lighter weight a lot of times. Usually the resistance provided by your own body is sufficient (e.g. *sit-ups*) and you will often find such exercises make up the final ten minutes of an aerobics class to tone muscles after cardiovascular work.

- **Flexibility** is the range of possible movements around a body joint or sequence of joints. For example, increased flexibility means that you come closer to being able to do the splits. Beware of thinking that practice will make perfect, because flexibility is affected by a number of other factors besides just working at it:

  –Your connective tissues, like ligaments and tendons, may be attached in ways that make flexibility more difficult.
  –The shape, size and arrangement of your bones will affect your flexibility
  –The bigger the muscle, the less room there is for free movement between the joints. Men tend to be less flexible than women, because they usually have bigger muscles.

  Obviously there is little you can do about these hereditary factors. However, you can really help your own flexibility through *yoga* exercises: sending mental energy from your centre to the joints you are stretching, and using your breath to ease you into increasingly exotic contortions.

Body language studies are beginning to prove that people with flexible, toned bodies are better able to project an image of self-confidence, so it may well be worth visiting a yoga class or two as part of your fitness programme.

- **Body Composition** is about how much excess fat you carry around. As you might expect, the less surplus fat you have, the fitter you are likely to be. Certain amounts of fat are critical – it is only the excess that you need to be concerned with. As with most aspects of your body, your fat stores are partially influenced by heredity.

Some people are more predisposed to fat deposits on thighs, while others find it settles on their tummies. And then there are those people who seem to have a natural fat repellent and remain lean despite doing no exercise at all. But do not be fooled into thinking that these people are necessarily fit merely because they have inherited a certain body type.

Males in general are composed of less fat than females. The percentage of fat distribution ranges from:

- 12–24% in men
- 19–30% in women

This is because females possess only minute quantities of the sex hormone *testosterone* that is so useful in making muscle. Again, do not be fooled, men are not inherently fitter than women; women need more fat reserves in order to ensure adequate energy for both the mother and the foetus in case of scarcity through pregnancy – a fantastic survival tactic.

Exercise can help in your battle against undesired fat in several ways:

- By strengthening and toning flabby muscles.
- By burning calories.
- By reducing your appetite (up to a point), as studies have shown that you eat more when you don't exercise than when you do.

Whatever your aim, start now

So, armed with this new knowledge about aspects of physical fitness, you are in a position to make decisions about the fitness programme that suits you. Be clear about your objectives. What do you want to be fit for?

- To climb stairs without losing your cool in the tube station.

- To increase your energy and capacity to achieve throughout the day.

- To lure a bedfellow, by slowly altering your body shape and self-image to become irresistible.

(Note: in modern slang the adjective 'fit' is used to describe someone sexually desirable – as in, 'Fwarrr – he/she's really fit'.)

- To build yourself up from puny to muscular – perhaps you want to feel that you are fit for a king or queen or perhaps you just want your size 12 clothes to fit.

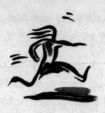

Health Clubs

As fitness is a long term venture, many people find that they need an extra motivating factor – the thought of getting into a bikini for your summer holiday may work for a couple of months, but will you continue your fitness programme come the autumn? Many find that money is the sustaining stimulant they require and therefore, if they pay to join a health club or gym, they have to go X times a week to make it worthwhile. Although this sounds good, our research has shown it to be a dangerous philosophy and you can no more buy dedication to fitness than you can order a completely new body from a catalogue.

Providing you make use of them, there are great advantages to belonging to a health club, primarily that everything is on tap, providing you with easy access to a vast range of activities for all round fitness and good health. The benefits of a good health club probably include:

- A gym with all the latest equipment
- A range of different classes (aerobics, circuit training boxercise, step, body biking, yoga etc.)
- A swimming pool
- Jacuzzi, sauna, steam room
- Hot showers (think of the money you'll save on bills) with shampoo, shower gel (more saving), hairdryers, body lotion, towels and machines to spin dry your swimming costume
- A shop in which to buy the latest designer sports gear
- A cafe/restaurant in which to indulge as a reward
- Sky TV (a real saving)
- Hairdressers, masseurs, beauticians, nutritionists etc
- Staff on hand to give help and advice
- Entrance forms for the marathon, just in case you get complacent

A tempting list, but before you fill a membership form and get your cheque book out (you could well find yourself spending something in the region of £650 annual subscription, plus a joining fee of little under £200), we will outline some of other activities that you are likely to get for your money. Remember, the best way to keep motivated and fit is to do something you actually enjoy.

The Gym

These days even the most modest gym will have an assortment of machines to give you a full workout. It is essential to get a professional to show you around and explain how to use them, in order that you work the right muscles in the right way and that you don't do yourself any harm. A good gym will give you a fitness assessment and draw up a programme designed to concentrate on the bits you particularly want/need to work on.

Unless you really want to work solely on *anaerobic* exercises (i.e. weights), we would advise a mixture of *CV training* (aerobic exercise) and *muscle toning activities*.

CV Equipment (Aerobic Exercise)

The machines that you are most likely to encounter are:

- *Treadmills* or running machines – you can programme these for different speeds and distances or times.

- *Training Bikes* – these can also be programmed for various settings with different 'hills', intensities and times. There are two types of bike – the upright and the recumbent, the latter giving more support to the back.

- *Steppers* – again these come in two main types – those which require small, fast steps and those where you push the steps right to the floor.

- *Rowing machines* – very effective for upper and lower body as long as you have a good technique. Technique is really very important on this piece of equipment, so do check with someone who knows. Basically the sequence of events should be: legs (push back), arms (pull), arms (release), legs (release), keeping your back straight and moving quickly backwards and slowly forwards.

- *Skywalkers* – these are cross country skiing simulators and use a large number of the muscles of the body. Many people fit a session at the gym in before work or in the lunch hour and want to pack as much work as they can into that time. This often means that a proper warm-up before the workout is dropped. While we would always advise that you don't leave out this important part of your session, if you insist upon leaving out a warm-up, then this machine will help warm up and stretch your whole body.

When working aerobically, be aware of these points:

- Always begin with a *warm-up* to prepare the body (particularly the heart) for the oncoming exertion and to get the blood flowing to the large muscles, particularly those of the legs. Literally, warming the muscles also means that they are better able to use

27

the oxygen in the blood, and gradually stretching them will lead to fewer strains and pulled muscles.

• During the stimulus period the primary activity should involve large muscles i.e. legs and arms.

• Activity should be continuous and rhythmic for periods of several minutes at a time.

• Activity should involve an increase in heart rate and some sweating (many of the machines mentioned will display your heart rate if you grab the bars with your hands).

• End each session with a *cool down*. Taper your exercise off slowly, as the body needs time for the heart rate, breathing and temperature to adjust. You also need to keep the blood flowing well, so it can remove the waste from the muscles and to bring new supplies of oxygen and glucose.

Try to exercise three to four times a week, starting with between 5 and 20 minutes per session and increasing gradually to about 90 minutes per week.

Weights (Anaerobic Exercise)

There are many different types of weights – *free weights* and *resistance machines*, *isolation* and *compound machines*. Again, you *must* ask advice and draw up a programme suited to your requirements.

As a general rule, try not to tire yourself out on the CV section of your workout to the extent that you have no energy left for muscle toning. Begin with the large muscle groups (shoulders, chest and back) which are often compound exercises, before moving on to the smaller isolation ones (biceps, triceps, quadriceps and hamstrings). For a toned stomach, the ultimate six-pack, the best exercises are sit-ups. There are resistance machines for abdominals, but they tend to put too much strain on the back.

Some pointers for muscle-building:

• Every contraction should be made through the full range of motion.

• An efficient way to improve muscle strength is through systematically overloading the muscle. Work with weights at a resistance of 6 RM (maximal repetitions) i.e. a weight so heavy that you can't lift it more than six times consecutively.

• Do three or four sets of each exercise with 5–10 minutes between sets for each muscle group.

• Try to train the muscles between once and three times a week, and not the same muscle groups on consecutive days.

This type of workout – on your own, in a gym – does require self-motivation. Whereas, in a class one is spurred on by others, and a public admission of defeat is something most of us try to avoid, at the gym, who's to know if you change the hill programme on the training bike from level 7 to level 2. What does it matter if you cut short your 20 minutes on the running machine? And do you really care if the computerised rower wins the race – just this once? Perhaps you do, in which case go for it! If not, perhaps you need a training partner to egg you on in an aggressive voice, to make sure you do your full quota of bicep curls, though they're bringing tears to your eyes, and to generate some 'healthy' competition. Do be careful though, because if you're not appreciating your partner's insistent commands as real concern for the size and shape of your muscles and a desire for you to realise your true potential, it may be the end of a beautiful friendship!

Classes

Like joining a gym, paying for a series of classes can often be a good way of motivating yourself to undertake exercise on a regular basis. Persuading a friend to accompany you will not only ease any apprehension, but also give you an added incentive; as you will probably feel bad about letting them down by failing to turn up.

Aerobics

What are they?

Classes consist of a 5–10 minute warm up and stretch, 20–30 minute CV work and 10–15 minutes toning and stretching.

Aerobics is, for us, the ultimate form of exercise, being demanding, tiring, satisfying, effective and, most importantly, good fun. It uses the whole body, improving stamina, flexibility and co-ordination.

Aerobics is a cardiovascular workout to cool music (hopefully), in which the routines get increasingly challenging as you progress from low impact beginner's classes to funky advanced sessions.

Although the routines are carefully choreographed, you are free to work as hard as you want. If struggling, you can march or walk through steps (rather than jog) and take out complicated arm movements while you find your feet. However tired or lost you might get, it is important to keep moving. If you suddenly stop, the result can be an accumulation or 'pooling' of blood in the veins, and this can mean that not enough blood gets back to the heart, making you feel dizzy or wobbly. So, march or walk on the spot – keep your feet going at all times. It is also important to drink plenty of water throughout the class to keep your body hydrated. If you don't, you may get a headache a couple of hours afterwards.

In your first aerobics class, nerves and self-consciousness may tempt you to stand at the very back. This has several disadvantages. Firstly, you will see very little of what the instructor is doing, which will make it very difficult to copy their routines. Secondly, directional changes – which are an integral part of any routine (in order to prevent undue stress to one side of the body) – often result in the back row becoming the front row before you've realised what's happening. We would therefore suggest that novices stand in the middle of a row, nearer the front than the back, to remain inconspicuous until you've got the hang of it. Try to avoid standing next to the over-zealous aerobics queens who will push each step to its limit, often at the expense of your personal space and your toes. As you get more confident, you can work your way forward to prime position next to the instructor. Generally, people are tolerant of newcomers and good-humoured about any mistakes you might make.

Learning a routine is deeply satisfying. In an 'add-on' class, separate sections are learnt and built up slowly to make the finished routine. Throughout these classes, you have the sense that you are working towards something rather than just exercising for its own sake. The greater the complexity of each individual section, the more your focus is drawn away from how hard you are working, as you concentrate from getting from A to B.

Aerobics Jargon

Aerobics has its own language. Be prepared to negotiate such moves as the *grapevine*, the *spotty dog*, the *box step* (or easy walk), the *washing machine*, *stars* and *half stars*, *hamstring curls*, *knee lifts* and *side steps*. Once you've learnt the basics, there are endless variations and instructors will often make up their own names for particularly complex steps. As long as you start with beginner's classes, you will not find yourself out of your depth and things will be explained as you go along.

What to wear

Lycra G-strings are not compulsory; ankle warmers and sweat-bands à la Bjorn Borg are definitely out. Basically, wear what you feel comfortable in – strip down from the big and baggy to the tiny and shiny as you get more confident. The only essential item is a good pair of trainers, which act as shock absorbers, protecting your joints. There is a huge choice of type and style of trainers and you should seek professional advice to find the most suitable pair for the type of activity you are interested in.

What not to wear

- *Excessive make-up*. Contrary to old-fashioned opinion, women *do* sweat. If you begin with full eye make-up, you are in danger of looking like a panda by the end of a tough class.
- *Hairspray*. There is little point going perfectly coiffured to a class, as you will end up with a soggy heap on top of your head. Tie your hair back; save the hairstyling for afterwards.
- *Perfume or after shave*. As you exercise you breathe deeply. You use full lung capacity and it is most unpleasant to breathe in strong artificial smells when you're desperate for fresh air.

Choosing an Instructor

A good instructor will vary the different sections, or change their order, so that you never do exactly the same routine and are constantly kept challenged and interested. Therefore, finding an inspirational instructor is vital. There are plenty of them, but discovering the ones for you is often a matter of trial and error.

Choosing a Class

Classes generally fall into two types: either dance based with inventive choreography or power based with simpler moves but more repetitions. You will probably be drawn to one or the other, but it is a question of experimenting with several different classes until you find the ones that you really enjoy. In the end it is enjoyment which will help sustain your commitment to a long-term programme.

Step Aerobics

Step aerobics often bears the brunt of cynical comments along the lines of 'Why don't you just walk up and down the stairs?' accompanied by incredulous laughter. Well, if you want to march up and down the stairs for 45 minutes, then do, but if you want a fun, challenging and satisfying work out, or you live in a bungalow, then you might find that 'step' is for you.

What are they?

On a very basic level, it is just stepping up and down on a 'board' (a platform 6–8 inches high). However, routines can get incredibly complicated, often with a lot of funky dance elements, and you can very easily find yourself facing completely the wrong direction, or tying your legs in knots, or just standing on top of your board dazed and confused. It is often bewildering to work out how an instructor got from A to B without falling over. But do not be put off!

If you are keen to succeed, you could practise at home on a plank of wood, balanced on telephone directories or on your coffee table. It is particularly important that you go back to the same class several times before you write this particular form of exercise off, as it can take a while to get the hang of.

Unlike straight aerobics, if you start on the wrong foot with step aerobics, or go the wrong way, it is very difficult to catch up and it's also more difficult to follow the general flow and direction of the class as the steps are small and contained. However, we have had great fun doing 'step', from the initial stages of getting it all wrong, to the immense satisfaction of getting a lot of it right. As with all these things, the more you have to concentrate on the steps, the less time you have to think how knackering it is.

Step Aerobics Jargon:

Some terms to watch out for are *basic step*, *turn step*, *T-step*, *Round the World*, *Superman*, *repeaters* and *Charleston*. As with aerobics, all these will be explained as you go along, provided you start at a beginner's level.

Warning:
Step aerobics does put pressure on your knees and, though a good technique will help prevent damage (most importantly always use a heel–toe action), if you have problems with your knee joints, this is probably not the activity for you.

Circuit Training

What is it?

Circuit training is a mixture of aerobic and muscle-toning exercises. Basically, you do a short aerobic workout and then a circuit of different activities with a specified amount of time on each station (or exercise), then more aerobics followed by another circuit, then more aerobics. This can happen any number of times depending on the class. You get a really excellent all round work out and can work to your own level on the stations. Because the time is limited on each activity (usually about 2 minutes), you will find that you can push yourself quite hard, particularly as the way they are spaced means that you won't be working the same muscle groups on consecutive stations.

Circuit Training Jargon

The sort of 'stations' you find are *press-ups*, *bicep curls* (different weights are usually provided), *tricep dips*, *lateral raises*, *crunchies*, *squat jumps*, *shuttle runs* and *star jumps*.

Choosing an Instructor

Do choose your instructor carefully as there are some frustrated sergeant majors about who bark instructions and order you to 'Come on!', rather than giving friendly encouragement. The masochists among you may welcome this approach, but it's not to everyone's taste.

There are many variations on the theme of exercising to music. As well as the old stalwarts; aerobics, step aerobics and circuit training, there are classes which concentrate on *Bums and Tums* or *Abs Fab*. There are *Stretch and Tone*, *Body Conditioning*, *Boxercise* and *Body Biking*, *Spin* and *Tri* classes. Also available are specialist classes for the over fifties and separate women's sessions.

It is good to go and be part of a group activity. Even if you decide that you don't particularly want to make friends with those who share your interest in fitness, their familiar faces will become strangely comforting after a while and the more often you go to the gym, the more it will start to feel like a second home.

Team Sports

Team games are sociable and can be great fun. There is also the added bonus of feeling obliged to turn up for the sake of your friends/team mates. These games can be taken as seriously as you like and can either involve a mess-around with a beach ball and a couple of jumpers in the park/your back garden, or joining the local team for weekly training and fixtures

Football

At the risk of sounding biased we would like it to be known that football is the best team game ever invented. A gentlemen's game played by yobs perhaps (as opposed to rugby which, the saying would have us believe, is a yob's game played by gentlemen) and it is certainly true that the off-pitch behaviour of many current football stars leaves a great deal to be desired. But the skill and invention displayed through a good flowing football match can take your breath away.

What You Need

Actually playing football – as opposed to watching it – if you're as four left-footed as we are, can be a demoralising experience. Therefore, you need to be armed with a sturdy sense of humour as well as a football (obviously), some jumpers that can serve as goalposts, and eight or nine friends if you're going to have a decent kick around. Choose these friends carefully. Many a firm friendship has collapsed at the local park as rivalries, usually well-concealed, come to the surface, and the competitive spirit gets the better of some people who forget they're meant to be enjoying themselves. Despite our lack of skill we probably burned up large amounts of calories just running madly after the ball and laughing at our own ineptitude so it's good exercise even if you can't do it.

The Rules

For those of you untutored in the rules of football the aim is to score goals by *passing* (to your team mates), *dribbling* (yuk), running with the ball and finally *shooting* past the opponent's goal-keeper hopefully into the net. You are not allowed to use your hands – hence *football* (which is a catchier name than footheadandchestball) – unless you are the goalkeeper when we advise *big* gloves otherwise it hurts.

If the other team have *possession*, you have to try and stop them scoring a goal by *marking* (putting them off, by getting between them and the ball), *tackling* (viciously, if you are undaunted by the risk of a red card) and occasionally, showing your knickers to the opposition – in the hope that this will distract them. This latter tactic has been known to work, but we suggest waiting until truly desperate before employing this tactic, as your credibility level tends to drop along with your trousers.

If such physical exertion doesn't appeal to you we have found that watching football can be in itself quite good exercise. Make sure you jump up and down a lot when someone scores or try and follow a goal with some celebratory dancing. If possible sit in a low chair and use your excitement to stand up every time the ball goes even vaguely near the net – you will find your thigh muscles work quite hard over 90 minutes. Use your arm muscles to gesture rudely at the referee when he makes bad decisions and try using the beer can you may, by chance, be drinking from as a weight for bicep curls through quiet stages of the match. When shouting at the TV, breathe properly and support your voice otherwise you may lose it – breathing exercises and a vocal warm-up may be helpful.

Finally, after the game, use your whole body to do impressions of some of the great moves and saves for a friend who missed the match itself. Through this, you not only provide a public service, recreating some of the magic for someone not lucky enough to catch it first time round, but you also give yourself a bonus mini-workout.

Cricket

If football strikes you as a tad too energetic, why not try cricket? Cricket is a game for those with time on their hands and a great deal of patience. Test matches – where one country plays another usually in a series of five tests – last for five days each, so its perhaps not the sport to choose if you're trying to hold down a 9-5 job too. But one-day matches are becoming more and more popular and you might find it's possible to fit one of those in at the weekend.

What You Need

You will need a cricket bat (traditionally made of willow wood), some jumpers to serve as wickets, and a very hard ball that can break your nose or knock you out if it hits you on the head so be careful. You may, as a novice, want to begin with a slightly less lethal tennis ball. You will also need some team mates and some opponents.

The Rules

Each team should take a turn (an *innings*) to *bowl* and *field* and then to *bat*. When fielding, the most important things to remember are: to try to catch any ball that comes near you (dive wildly towards it if need be); to stay awake, even if the ball has come nowhere near your position in the outfield for hours, and *never* to throw like a girl when returning the ball to the bowler, or indeed when bowling itself. 'Girls' throw underarm and this is just not 'cricket'. This makes life a little difficult for those of us who never managed the cool overarm technique at school but try to battle on regardless. Your aim is to stop the batsperson scoring *runs* (hitting the ball with such strokes as a *pull*, a *hook*, a *cover drive*, a *grubber*, a *Chinese cut*, a *late cut*, a *square cut*, and running between the *wickets* (jumpers) while the ball is returned to the bowler), so the quicker you field the better.

Keeping score in cricket is quite complicated – on TV the commentator will talk about the bowler's figures and numbers which sound a bit like measurements, so you could be forgiven for thinking there is some kind of fashion show occurring. In fact, it is worth understanding the system here, perhaps – if other reasons escape you – because we have been reliably informed that it is sexy to know about cricket.

Very briefly, a bowler bowls six balls per over; if no runs are scored it is called a *maiden over*; the bowler's figures are expressed as I (or 2 or 3 – however many batspeople have been got out) **for**, say, **93** (or 45 or 2 – however many runs have been scored). It's as simple as that. When batting, try not to score a *duck* (0 runs), get *lbw*, *caught* or *run out*, but score 4's and 6's by hitting the ball to the boundary or beyond and make a *century* of runs if you possibly can. If all else fails shout 'Howzzat!' a lot at the umpire, look forward to the civilised breaks for lunch and tea and unpack that sturdy sense of humour to make sure you have a good day.

There is something very calming about watching cricket if you don't fancy playing, and it may be a good opportunity to practise some yoga techniques and breathe yourself into a state of pure relaxation as the hours pass by.

Rugby

If you are a braver sort of person, undaunted by the prospect of (often very large) people charging at you and trying to mow you down, perhaps rugby is your thing. Rugby is a contact sport, where tackling involves shouldering people to the floor, or wrapping yourself around their moving feet to trip them up. Anything that would get you a red card in football is OK in rugby – including handling the ball – but the line is drawn at biting bits of opponent's ears off, so not quite anything goes. A rugby ball is a strange shape, designed to make it difficult to anticipate the direction of its bounce and therefore you must be prepared to scramble after it and hurl yourself on top of it. Leave your dignity at home and know that your clothes will be filthy if you've played properly.

The Rules

The aim is to score tries by putting the ball down over the other team's *try line* (indicated by those trusty jumpers if you're at your local park) and then to convert that *try* into more points by kicking the ball over the goal between the posts (the jumpers are struggling here but never mind). You need to use your team mates to kick to or to hand pass to (where the ball must be thrown backwards) and hopefully to progress further and further towards the try line. On the way you take part in *tackles*, *line-outs* and *scrums* where people bundle together extremely closely and pull on each other's shorts. It's a strange but wonderful game, and if the thought of it scares you slightly then just think how many calories you could burn up by running screaming away from all the attacks aimed at you. Again, you don't have to be good to get a good work out.

These three team sports are traditionally men's games but there is nothing to stop women playing. Your local club team will almost certainly have a women's section and you might be surprised at its standard, so if you're serious about playing, go along and find out how to join in. For those of you who want a way to add variety to your fitness programme, an afternoon spent having a go at any of these games can be very worthwhile.

Just as traditional men's games needn't be restricted to men, playing traditional women's games are also open to all.

Netball

There are mixed as well as single sex leagues and many colleges and corporate businesses are developing mixed teams as part of their 'bonding' programmes. Cute little netball skirts are optional though you may discover they help the bonding process. Vests with big capital letters explaining your position (eg C = Centre, W = Wing Defence, GA = Goal Attack) are helpful as each position is restricted to certain areas of the court.

What You Need

Although netball courts are readily available in all good school playgrounds, if you are making your own you will need to bring your entire jumper collection to mark out all the zones and to construct two netball posts with baskets.

You will need six friends to make up your team and seven enemies to fight against. You must all be prepared to leap about like spring lambs, be bouncy, quick off the mark and able to play in short, sharp bursts.

The Rules

The ball is moved down the court from player to player using *chest passes*, *shoulder passes* and *bounce passes* until it reaches the *Goal Attack* or *Goal Shooter* whose job it is to *shoot* the ball through the opponent's basket. When passing, careful footwork is important: you are only allowed to take two steps on receiving the ball and then have three seconds in which to pass it. Women have the upper hand here as men tend to get confused with basketball in which you are allowed to run with the ball, as long as you bounce it. Men, with generally added height have their day when it comes to goal scoring.

Obviously, if you are defending you must do your best to intercept the ball and stop goals being scored by jumping up and down in front of the shooter. You can employ fair means or foul to distract their concentration, as long as you are standing three feet away.

If someone does a Bad Thing (like touching or barging) he must be punished and stand beside the person he has fouled with his head hung in shame while the fouled player takes a penalty pass.

The game is divided into quarters of either 15 or 20 minutes, but obviously you can set your own time scale according to your requirements.

Hockey

Despite the 'jolly hockey sticks' image, hockey is very much a unisex sport. It is brutal.

What You Need

Do not attempt to play without shin pads, gum shield and, if you are in goal, all the protection you can lay your hands on. If you haven't got the proper gear for this, wrap yourself in a duvet (which will also give you your own private sauna while others run around the pitch) and wear a cycling helmet. You will also need a hockey stick and a hard ball and serious women's teams also seem to find it necessary to wear bandannas.

The Rules

The rules are similar to football, but you are not allowed to put your body between the ball and an opposing player as this counts as an *obstruction* and you must always use your hockey stick rather than your foot or head (ouch!).

You are allowed to 'roll' substitutes on and off the pitch whenever you need to, as long as the number of players on the pitch remains constant.

You use *stick stops*, *reverse stick stops*, *reverse dodges*, *right hand dodges* and *ball circling* to manoeuvre the ball from one end of the pitch to the other, and then shoot at the goal.

If you're short on fitness-minded friends, team sports are difficult, but you can surely find one ally. Have a **tennis** knockabout, a sweaty game of **squash**, or, if you're worried by the risk of ball injury, shuttlecocks and **badminton** racquets might provide the answer. Sex is also a great calorie burner. Do not just lie back and think of England, be as athletic as you can, as often as possible.

Any sports/games which get you out and about and raise your heart rate will be beneficial, but don't be lured into thinking that every sport is physically good for you. Darts, cards, tiddlywinks and the like will not bring you the body of your dreams.

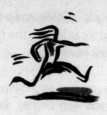

Things You Can Do On Your Own

Perhaps all this talk of group exercise is scaring you off a bit and what you really want to do is work on your own, as and when you feel like it.

Fitness Videos

If this is the case, then you may wish to consider a fitness video to bring a class into your very own living room – with people who wear the same outfits every time, always stand in the same places and never even bat an eyelid when you get it all horribly wrong.

There is an enormous range of such videos on the market, made by all sorts of people from supermodels to soap stars, sports personalities to gracefully ageing celebrities. The choice can be overwhelming, and although we have tried out a number, we have only scratched the surface of what's available. In our experience, picking a role model is a fairly good way of choosing a video. For example, if you would like a figure like Cindy Crawford's, then the notion that doing the exercises she does will result in achieving her body shape, might keep you going for quite a while. At some stage you might have to come to terms with the fact that you and Cindy were made from different moulds. Hopefully by that stage you will have increased your level of fitness, feel much better about yourself and be prepared for you and her to differ.

For men, fitness video role models are rather scarce – would you like to be a Jeremy Guscott or a Mr. Motivator? Many men do seem to be drawn to the likes of Cindy Crawford, but this is a different sort of motivating factor (and perhaps a different sort of exercise).

Ideally you should try a few out before you buy one, hiring them from video rental shops or libraries to find the sort of thing you want.

Muscle Toning Videos

• *The Stretch* – Sharron Davies
  Concentrates on muscle toning and stretching, also includes a long section on nutrition and beauty that you probably wouldn't watch very often.

• *For a Better Bust* – Rosemary Conley

From her *Top to Toe* collection this video, as you might expect, is about upper body training. Therefore you would probably want to use it in conjunction with one or more of her other numerous videos to ensure 'Top to Toe' fitness (the money making point, we suspect, of the collection).

- *Britt Fit* – Britt Eckland
  Coyly aimed at 'women of a certain age'. Concentrates on muscle toning rather than CV training. The exercises are much the same as you find on all these videos, giving your body a good all round workout. Unfortunately there is nothing remotely dynamic about it and the voice over is out of sync and terribly uninspiring. Having learnt the exercises you might be better off devising your own workout.

Aerobic Videos

- *The Y Plan Series*
  If it is an aerobics video you want (which will include a muscle toning section as well) you are similarly spoilt for choice. We found *The Y Plan* series to be very good, straightforward, informative and unpretentious (a rare thing where these videos are concerned). As well as providing good, short but effective workouts at different levels, *The Y Plan Physical* also has a fitness assessment section so you can monitor your progress regularly. (Note that Anthea Turner mysteriously disappears after her

assessment, while Jeremy Guscott takes part in both workouts. Maybe she didn't like the outfits...)

- *Ease into Fitness* – Diana Moran
  The Green Goddess encourages you to *Ease into Fitness* and the emphasis really is on EASE – in fact, she suggests that the first time you just watch! We never once broke into a sweat, despite promises of progressively harder aerobics, and we had to pinch ourselves to stay awake between movements in the 'Pulse Raiser'. At one point the Green Goddess cries 'It's a party!' which left us staring at the television open mouthed. The video case boasts an alluring list of music including numbers such as 'Bend Me, Shape Me', 'Celebration' and 'La Bamba' – so if it's hard-core dance music you want, this is definitely not for you. Again, there is a pretty comprehensive muscle toning section, but again, you can do this yourself.

- *10 Minute BLTs* – Mr. Motivator
  Offers a good workout for bums, legs and tums, with a fat burning section (rather repetitive) and endless warm ups in case you are not doing the whole video in one go. Filmed in Tobago, this video made us think that actually it was purely an excuse for Mr. M. to go on a great holiday with three people he obviously likes flirting with. They're all having such a great time, laughing and 'whooping' throughout and don't even flinch when Mr. Motivator puts his hands on their bums – oh sorry, their gluteals.

While we agree with the general philosophies that our ridiculously clad video leader spouts and appreciate the atmosphere of fun, I think if we had to go through this too many times, we would end up hating them all, resenting the insistent commands to 'Smile' throughout and not doing the exercise. Also, some of the exercises are demonstrated and then you need to switch off the video and do a few sets on your own, which might annoy you, having shelled out the cash.

• *The Body Workout* – Elle Macpherson
The best of the ones we tried is Elle Macpherson's *The Body Workout*, in which Elle's personal trainer, Karen Voight, takes you through a circuit of three aerobic sessions interspersed with muscle toning exercises, with a warm up and cool down at either end. The fact that the workout is divided into these alternating sections means that you don't tire, physically or psychologically, of one thing or the other, but can keep the intensity going for the whole programme.

A straightforward workout, very suitable for men as well as women (we say this because it is un-dancey rather than because it's got Elle Macpherson in it), with the opportunity to make exercises harder (by using weights) if required. We found it quite comforting that, though she may have a fantastic body, Elle is, by her own admission, a bit uncoordinated and really does not look a natural in the aerobics scene. Her comments sound rather scripted and cheesy, but there aren't many of them and probably wouldn't figure highly on the irritation scale.

- *Cher Fitness – A New Attitude* – Cher
  Cher's step video has a very good aerobic section with different levels suggested (one poor woman does the entire class without a step and another never gets to use her arms) and quite challenging choreography. The floor exercises are likewise very good and the whole video will probably provide you with a challenge for quite some time. However, you do have to put up with Cher singing along to her own songs, which is too much for some people.

(If you like the idea of step aerobics and are prepared to buy your own step (about £50), then this can be a very good way of exercising at home. You can make do with a much smaller space than straight aerobics and you can get a very effective, if rather unimaginative, workout by stepping up and down whilst watching television – which kills two birds with one stone and takes your mind off the effort of exercising.)

The thing about all these videos is that they never change, which results in a serious boredom factor. Once you have noticed one slightly irritating characteristic (a particularly nauseating line of encouragement, or someone in the back row going wrong), repeated viewing can turn it into a source of extreme aggravation, leading you to shout abuse or hurl things at the television. When we reached this stage, we decided not to bother with the video any more. We know the routines, so we can use our own choice of music (and its not often that we reach for 'Celebration' or the like) and modify, or even improve on, the routines to keep ourselves amused and constantly challenged.

If, like us, you are (or think you might be) a keen aerobics-goer, you still might like to have one of these videos as a reserve for those occasions when other commitments mean you are unable to get to your favourite class.

Running

As CV training goes, running is highly effective and very accessible; you are rarely restricted by the weather or your surroundings. You won't waste any time getting to and from the gym (unless you want to run round a track) and you can fit it into your day free from timetables or lane restrictions. The only thing you will have to spend money on is a good pair of running shoes Although running is a natural activity, there are some points to be aware of to avoid injury and orthopaedic problems. The most important is not to run on your toes. The movement should be heel–toe: land on the heel and push off from the toe, and try to keep your feet pointing as directly forwards as possible, even if you walk with your toes pointed out slightly. This (and good shoes) will help prevent shin splints – a very common complaint in many runners, in which sharp pains are felt in the front of the lower leg.

Another factor to consider is the type of surface you run on. It is best to avoid very hard surfaces such as Tarmac and concrete, and try to run on grass or dirt paths. If you run on a track, make sure you change direction (clockwise/anticlockwise) regularly. If you always run in the same direction, the muscles on the inside leg may well develop differently from those on the outside leg, leading to problems when the muscles are forced to compensate on the straight.

Things to bear in mind:

- As with all the exercise ideas we have put forward, a warm up is essential before you run, preparing your body for what's to come to prevent stress, damage and injury.
- Once you have got going, don't feel that you have to run the whole time. If you intersperse running with short periods of walking, you will probably find that you are able to do more total work.
- You should ensure that you are working to the level you want by checking your heart rate according to these training zones:

> 60 – 70% of your maximum heart rate (HR)
> = FAT BURNING
>
> 70 – 80% of your max HR
> = MODERATE/INTENSE TRAINING
>
> 80 – 85 % of your max HR
> = INTENSE TRAINING
>
> Your maximum heart rate is roughly 220 beats per minute minus your age.
>
> • At the end of your run, don't just stop – bring your heart rate down slowly and stretch the muscles out.

Warning:

We must stress that you should introduce an exercise programme like this *gradually*. If you set off on your first outing to run for an hour, you will probably fail and get disheartened, or injure yourself. Be realistic and increase your session (warm up, run and cool down) over time to an hour three times a week. In the long 'run' you may discover a *Forrest Gump*ian gift and find that you just can't stop.

Swimming

Swimming is often cited as being one of the best forms of exercise. Unlike running, swimming exercises the upper and lower body and, perhaps the best thing about it is that you are supported by the water. There is none of the constant stress placed on the knees and ankles in many other forms of exercise – the water provides the resistance and the support. Because of this, swimming is very good if you are recovering from an injury, have back or other orthopaedic problems or if you are pregnant. Likewise, if you are overweight, this activity is very good to start with, as it will not put strain on your joints.

People often think that they aren't working hard enough when swimming – perhaps because the normally perceptible signs of exertion, such as sweating and shortness of breath, are not quite so evident. So, knowledge of the training zones could be very beneficial here. If you want to do a structured, intensive training session you are best advised to join a club where you will be given training programmes and can carry them out in private sessions, as it is often quite difficult to get a proper workout in public pools. Negotiating your 64 lengths can be a hazardous procedure, involving dodging unsavoury floating plasters, swimming round slow coaches in the fast lane (who take great offence if it is suggested that they might be better suited to the medium or – God forbid – slow lanes), negotiating elderly back-stokers (who, unwittingly, swim diagonally across the pool) and avoiding children desperate to dive bomb you. There are different sessions at most pools: lengths only, over 25s, women only etc and it is a good idea to find the one which holds the least deterrents.

Aqua Aerobics

Many pools also have aqua aerobics classes, and these sessions are fantastic for people interested in doing something more varied with their time in the water than just swimming up and down. Aqua aerobics – unless it is a 'deep water' class – take place at the shallow end of the pool so you never need go out of your depth. This may encourage non-swimmers to take part and perhaps overcome some of their fear of the water by spending a session in the pool, hopefully having fun, without feeling like a failure because they aren't swimming.

As with straightforward swimming, aqua aerobics is kinder to joints than other sports. The water supports your body weight and provides resistance to work against – like using weights. So again, if you are pregnant, injured or overweight this may be a sensible place to start your exercise programme.

Most classes will consist of a warm-up, a CV workout and a toning section, with the instructor leading the class from the poolside. Music makes your time in the water more fun, although the speaker systems in pools usually sound a bit dodgy. If you are self-conscious about revealing yourself in a swimming costume – and we must all have felt this at some point – try to remember that once you have taken the plunge and are in the pool the entire session takes place under the water where no-one can see you. You will get a good work out, almost in private. If you do feel self-conscious, place a towel by the side of the pool to wrap yourself in afterwards and there is nothing to worry about.

Cycling

Another excellent CV activity, and one that doesn't stress the joints as much as running. It is also, of course, a useful way to get around – quicker than running and of more use than swimming (unless you live by a lake or on an island, in which case you could swim to work). Cycling can help you beat the traffic, is environmentally friendly, keeps you fit and tones those thigh muscles.

Dancing

You don't have to be a dedicated ballet dancer to enjoy the benefits of dancing. Tap dancing apparently gives you the best legs of all, but if you don't fancy yourself as a Fred Astaire or a Ginger Rogers, a good sweaty dance at a club constitutes an effective CV workout. You can, of course, do this at home: find some funky music, turn it up really loud and anything goes. Remove all mirrors and other people from the room and become Coco from *Fame*, John Travolta in *Saturday Night Fever*, Robbie Williams or a Spice Girl for 20 minutes. The lack of structure is unimportant – just raise your pulse, sweat and have a laugh.

In fact, if the dancing doesn't inspire you, just do the laughing. A good 20 minute giggle session gives your face and stomach an excellent workout and burns calories.

Other Ideas

Household and garden chores can also help keep you in shape, particularly if you make yourself aware of the muscle groups and use them effectively. For example, why not combine the hoovering (or mowing the lawn) with some lunges, working the quadriceps, or get at that dusty top shelf with some squat jumps, or take time to work the backs of the thighs while ironing. Pulling stubborn weeds out of the garden can be very good for the upper body and, providing you have enough weeds, you can work a full range of muscles. The use of garden shears is very beneficial for the pectorals; make a roux sauce or whisk some eggs for a good arm workout, or use those heavy bags of shopping as weights, doing a set of bicep/tricep curls on the way from the car to the house...

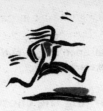

Muscle Toning Exercises

You may wish to combine cardiovascular activities with some muscle toning work. The diagrams below show exercises that will tone the main muscle groups.

You should be aiming to do two or three sets of 20 repetitions of each exercise. When different levels of intensity are shown, begin on the easiest and, over the next few months, when all three sets are within your capabilities, move up to the next.

Likewise with weights, begin with one pound or none at all and move up when you feel ready. Where progressive levels are not shown, it is a question of slowly increasing the repetitions you do over time. Don't push yourself too far, because overdoing it on one day can put you out of action for the rest of the week. Little and often is always better than big bursts which take weeks to recover from.

Arms

In all these exercises, don't 'lock out' the arms (ie don't straighten the arms completely).

Press ups – working the chest and biceps

Box position
Hands a bit more than shoulder width apart, back straight, stomach pulled in. Keep the movement slow and controlled, don't lock out the elbows on the way up and don't collapse on the floor on the way down.

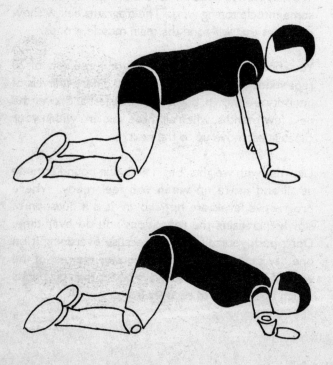

3/4 position
Keep your body in a straight line from knees to shoulders.

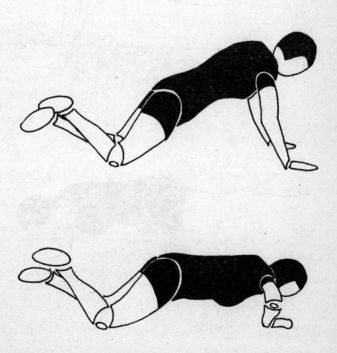

Full position
Keep your body in a straight line from heels to shoulders.

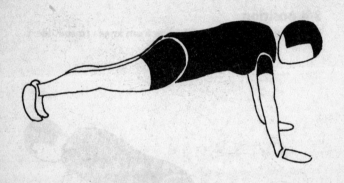

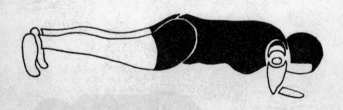

Triceps

(With weights [1lb - 5lbs] or tins)

Keep your elbows close to the body and pointing up to the ceiling.

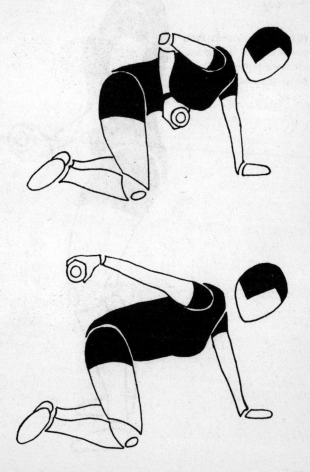

Bicep curls

**Control the movement
on the way down as well
as the way up. Tuck the
elbows into the sides of
the body.**

**(Keep your knees soft,
pelvis tucked under and
stomach pulled in. Don't
tense the neck.)**

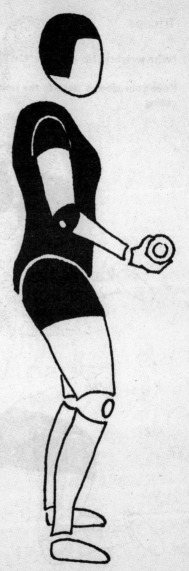

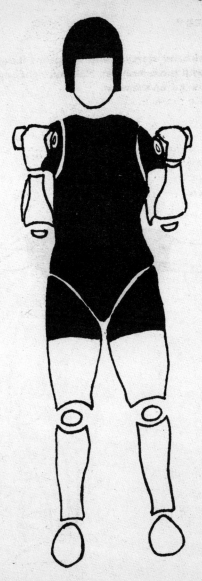

Pec-Decs

Rotate the arms starting with the palms facing out and finishing with them facing in. Maintain right angles at the elbow – don't drop the arms.

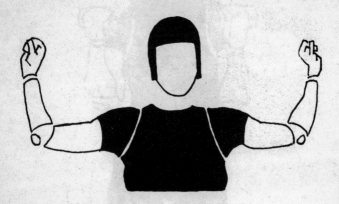

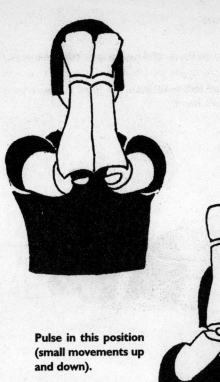

Pulse in this position (small movements up and down).

Legs and Bums

In all these exercises be careful not to lock out the knees.

Push hips forward and lead with the heel. Support your weight on the front hand.

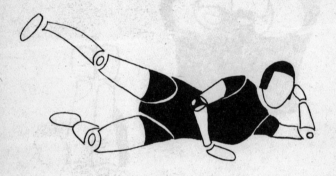

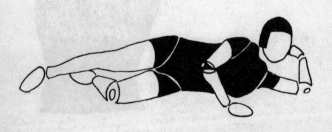

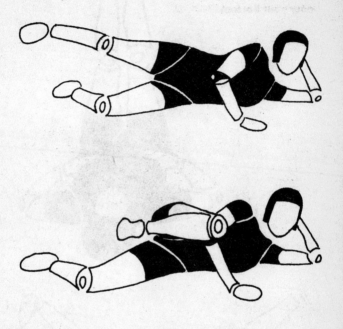

Always control the movement, don't kick the leg.

Point toes on the way up and flex them back on the way out. Keep stomach muscles tight. If you find you can't keep the small of the back on the floor, place your hands under your bottom.

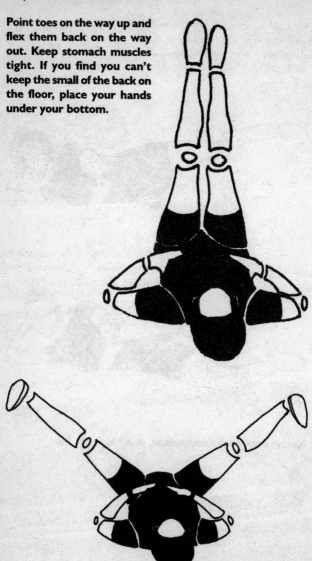

Use the upper and lower abdominals to bring your shoulders and knees towards each other.

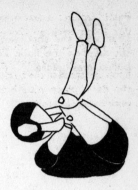

Sit Ups

A small movement, tilt the pelvis and pull the stomach muscles down to the floor. The hands support the head but must not pull on the neck. If you don't need the support place your fingers at the temples.

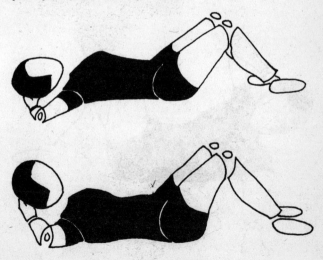

Obliques

Lead with the shoulder, *not* the elbow. Keep the other shoulder on the floor. Pelvis tilted and stomach muscles pulled in as before.

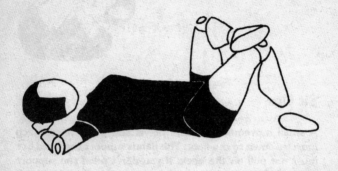

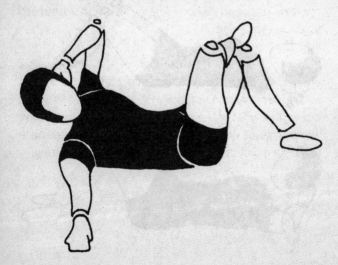

Healthy Eating

Eating is one of the great pleasures in life, but for many it is often difficult to eat moderately and sensibly, and eating healthily may seem unappealing or impossible. Perhaps you are exercising so that you can continue to eat whatever you like without gaining weight. Nonetheless, we would stress that a healthy, balanced diet will keep your body happy, and, along with your exercise plan, you will be firing on all cylinders and will look and feel great.

As a nation we eat far too much of all the things that are worst for us: convenience has replaced nutrition as the most important factor. We need to regain some interest in what makes up the food we eat and some knowledge of what our bodies require. We aim here to give a quick guide to the basics of healthy eating.

Fat

The word that sends shivers through many of us, making us vow to rid it from our lives through existing on Rivita and running. But **fat provides energy and, in the right amounts, is essential**. However, excess fat is stored in layers beneath the skin and is therefore what we want to avoid.

There are two types of fats:

- Saturated – mainly animal in origin
- Unsaturated – from vegetable sources

Of our general fat intake, the proportions of saturated:unsaturated fats is 75%:25%. Too much *saturated* fat increases your calorie count, so aim to reduce your fat intake as a whole by 25%, and subsequently reverse the proportions of saturated: unsaturated fat consumption.

Some pointers:

- Use polyunsaturated cooking oils and spreads
- Avoid red/preserved meat and sausages
- Eat more fish and chicken
- Eat more beans (pulses), grains and seeds
- Use skimmed/semi-skimmed milk

Generally a diet that is high in whole, unrefined foods and low in manufactured foods will be about 25% lower in fat than the average British diet.

Carbohydrate

Also vital for energy, this is found in bread, potatoes, pasta, rice, sweets and sugar. Try to go for *starch*, which is a *complex carbohydrate* (a mix of simple sugars that break down steadily to provide energy) found in wholemeal bread, cereals, potatoes, pasta and pulses. If you are exercising regularly, it is essential to have a diet high in carbohydrate for your energy supply.

Many people avoid carbohydrates as 'fattening', but this is not so: it is not the baked potato which will make you put on weight, but the butter you spread on top of it; nor is it the pasta, but the creamy sauce in which it is covered.

Protein

Important for the growth and repair of tissue. Although red meats and dairy products are particularly high in protein, you would do better to get your quota from fish, white meat and vegetables, which are not so high in fat.

Fibre

Essential for healthy bowels and not present in many pre-packed foods. Yet another reason for eating fresh fruit and vegetables, wholemeal bread, rice and beans.

Sugar

Good for us in small quantities. Unless you are going to run a marathon, climb a mountain or do anything else requiring an enormous amount of energy, the sugar that exists naturally in foods should be enough. Remember: excess sugar = excess calories. Try to avoid refined sugar (chocolate, sweets, cakes etc) and replace it with natural sources such as fruit.

Salt

Something else to cut down on. It can cause high blood pressure and is associated with strokes. Manufactured food is generally incredibly high in salt, so eating fresh food is an easy way to reduce our intake. Also avoid adding too much salt when cooking — perhaps try herbs and spices instead.

Water

An essential part of the body tissue and vital for health and physical performance. Of course, pure water is best for you but, failing that, try to avoid sugary drinks and those with added colouring.

Caffeine

A central nervous system stimulant which raises the blood sugar level very quickly, giving a short-lived feeling of vitality. Chemically, it speeds up mineral loss and produces acid in the stomach, and in the long term can cause chronic insomnia, anxiety, depression and gastric irritation.

Alcohol

Enters the blood stream quickly, and our faithful bodies try to use it as energy. However, like too much sugar, it can't make use of it all, especially as you're probably sitting down (using one calorie per minute).

Vitamins and Supplements

Vitamins and minerals are important for good health, but if we eat a balanced diet of fresh and whole foods, we shouldn't need supplements. Any extra will only be peed out – truly money down the drain.

For a balanced diet, try to eat your quota from these five groups:

- *CEREAL GROUP*
  At least four portions a day.
  Wholegrain bread, rice, pasta, potatoes and breakfast cereals.

- *FRUIT AND VEGETABLES GROUP*
  At least three portions a day.
  Include carrots (vitamin A) several times a week and green vegetables (for folic acid) daily.

- *MEAT, NUTS AND PULSES GROUP*
  Two portions a day.
  Nuts, pulses and grains provide essential fatty acids (EFAs), calcium, vitamins and fibre. Fish also provide EFAs and Vitamin D, and red meat is a good source of iron, but high in saturated fat.

- *MILK GROUP*
  One portion a day (1/2 pint of milk).

Milk, yoghurt, cheese – high in protein, calcium and vitamin A (but also saturated fat). If you don't like milk products, you can get these from dark green vegetables, dried fruit, crushed and baked seeds and soya.

- **FLUID GROUP – 6 – 7 glasses a day.**

Incorporating all these food groups into your diet in roughly the right quantities *is* possible, but take it slowly. If you completely change your diet overnight, you will probably last a couple of days, resent it and revert to your old ways. Start by adding things rather than by denying yourself the things you like most, and you will find that your body will develop a taste for the good things.

Maybe this sounds implausible, but we know it to be a fact. We were both confirmed chocoholics – thought we couldn't go into a shop without buying a chocolate bar (unless, of course, it wasn't that sort of shop) and didn't really think carefully about what we ate. Now we rarely eat chocolate and would never buy it as a matter of course and this has happened quite naturally. Of course we still get cravings, and we do respond to them, but they don't happen often, as we have got out of the habit of having chocolate every day.

You don't get fit and healthy by being a martyr – from abstaining from anything that isn't 100% fat free and packed with vitamins. Subscribe to the old adage 'everything in *moderation*', sometimes you need to treat yourself. But over the course of several months, your body will begin to view treats differently and will be drawn more to those things that are positively good for you.

Diets (*boo, hiss*)

Playing on our unhappy predilection towards guilt has become the diet ad-man's most effective and successful tactic. We feel guilty about eating; we feel guilty about not conforming to desirable body shapes; we often feel guilty about not being perfect. We spend millions of pounds on special foods, devices, magazines, and slimming clubs – many of them medically endorsed – in an effort to cure what we have been encouraged to view as unsightly fatness.

Too much body weight – obesity – is considered a disease and is medically linked to heart problems, high blood pressure, gallstones, diabetes and arthritis. But studies have never conclusively proved that the weight itself is the cause of such problems. Apparently it could actually be the result of the bad diet and the lack of exercise and physical fitness which often accompanies obesity. Weighing more than 'the average' does not necessarily mean you are more prone to any illness. Heavier than average people can be as healthy as anyone else, as long as they eat the right foods and keep themselves fit. In fact, they are probably more likely to be healthy than severely underweight people, particularly those who use low-calorie diets to secure their weight loss.

The disadvantages of low-calorie diets

There are some worrying facts about low-calorie diets that it is as well to be aware of in case you are thinking of embarking on one. The most helpful thing to advise is probably 'Don't bother'. Over a five-year period 98–99% of women who diet regain their weight. In fact 90% regain more than they lost, meaning that dieting can actually make you fatter in the long run.

These figures sound extraordinary, but putting weight back on after dieting is actually quite understandable. It has nothing to do with your own lack of will power and should never be viewed as some kind of failure. In self-preservation our bodies adapt to a low-calorie food intake in ways that are beyond our control. It does not matter how strict you are with yourself or how firm your resolve is, your body will make it very difficult to maintain weight loss over a period of time.

Therefore unless food intake reduction is coupled with a fitness programme of regular exercise, there really seems to be very little point in dieting. You are fighting a losing battle. For each month you continue eating the same low number of calories your rate of weight loss is usually cut in half. This is because your body adjusts to a lower calorie intake and becomes more efficient at using and storing calories. The calories you burn to keep your basic body functions going (basic metabolism) can decrease by as much as 30%. When you stop starving yourself you replace and often exceed your original weight quickly – and mostly in the form of fat – because you have forced your body to become more efficient, burning off fewer calories immediately and storing more fat for later use.

As well as being ineffective in the long-term, low-calorie dieting is an unhealthy way of life. Many slimming diets recommend restricting yourself to between 700 and 1000 calories per day but The World Health Organization (WHO) defines starvation as a calorie intake of less than 1000 calories a day. Whether self-imposed, or forced by situation, starvation is starvation. Starvation causes listlessness, apathy, lethargy, headaches, dizziness, light-headedness and depression.

If, for any extended period of time you have a calorie intake of less than the WHO's approximate recommendation of 2,200 calories per day, then it's probable you'll experience some or all of the above symptoms. You are probably lacking necessary nutrients and you'll almost certainly be uninspired by the idea of a good work out – the thing which is most likely to help you lose weight – because you'll have no energy. You are not doing yourself any favours.

Sensible Dieting

If you really feel you need to go on a diet, make sure you get fit at the same time and don't reduce your daily calorie intake by more than 500. Give yourself a realistic time limit to work within. Don't expect overnight miracles. If you take things slowly you could have considerably altered your body shape by this time next year and have gradually altered your way of life so that any changes are long-term and for real. A great body is within everyone's grasp as long as you realise that a great body means toned and fit, not skin and bone.

Anorexia nervosa

Beware of anorexic tendencies. It is good to be honest with yourself about obsessions and try to force yourself out of any potentially dangerous thought processes before they take a grip. This is never easy, but if you can nip things in the bud using sense and reason, you can avoid years of suffering.

Anorexia is a tragic modern illness and, while every case is different, anorexics display common patterns. Anorexia is often seen as an attempt to assert control over life through control over the body and a heroic display of self-restraint and self-discipline; perhaps an unconscious cry for help, for attention; perhaps an escape or denial of adulthood. Always a betrayal of terribly low self-esteem and of epic emotions which for some reason find no other escape route and get turned in on themselves.

Anorexia nervosa is a mental illness, but it is also a social disease. While we live in a society that focuses on exteriors and facades, and suggests through its advertising that conforming to stereotyped body images of perfection can result in happiness and power, then we will all continue to be at risk.

For further information, read *Conquering Anorexia* by Clare Lindsay, also published by Summersdale.

The Perils of Advertising

Life can be cruel to those with the best intentions and it's as well to be aware of some of the booby traps that may lie ahead. Forewarned is forearmed.

Our society often makes things very difficult for the average person – particularly for the average person trying to look after him or herself and get fit. Stereotypes are everywhere and media role models still all seem to be about fairly plastic surface beauty. Pamela Anderson and three square inches of Lycra is the Playboy bunny brought to life, hopping along a beach near you. Jean-Claude Van Damme, the Muscles from Brussels, equipped with the latest hi-tech killing machine, is a walking, talking cartoon superhero. Little stick people creak up and down catwalks around the developed world wearing bin-liners that cost thousands and real fur dyed and treated to make it appear fake. Things are warped.

You turn on the TV during advert time and a beautiful woman is in the bath with a chocolate flake. She and the flake are making love. The woman has a look of wanton abandonment and she has forgotten that if you leave taps running your bath overflows and your flat floods – facts which we in the real world are made to feel slightly foolish for worrying about. Why aren't men up in arms about adverts like these? Do they not mind being so easily replaced by pieces of crumbly, flaky milk chocolate?

While the woman takes a bath, the male chocolate eating equivalent drives a truck. Long distance. He wears black leather and faded denim; he has no worries, girls will fall at his feet. He takes big man-sized mouthfuls of his big man-sized chocolate bar and he nods with utter fulfilment, he has eaten chocolate; his life is complete.

Such images are powerful. Even drinking a particular brand of coffee can help you to relationship bliss with the man of your dreams, as if two people needed nothing more in common than this in order to secure life happiness. It is all rubbish, of course. But however strong and independent-minded we may think we are there is something all-pervasive about these advertising suggestions.

A long-term fitness routine, which requires constant input over many months, seems like a waste of time when the answer to all life's problems can be bought over the counter of your local newsagent. It takes great determination to rise above the multimillion-pound advertising industry and be sensible about what you need to do, and to eat, and to be. Try to remember that advertising often makes your life more difficult than it already is. Cream cakes for example are not 'Naughty but Nice' They are just 'Nice'. Have one if you want. Have an affair with a flake once in a while too. Balance is everything.

The 'Naughty' part of that particular advertising campaign betrays one of the most worrying prevalent social attitudes. Eating food – or more particularly not eating food – seems to have become so tied up with our perception of morality that much time will be needed to sort out the resulting mess. You hear people claiming that they have been 'good' because they had no breakfast or 'really bad' because they had pudding. Good and bad? It is ridiculous. Get some perspective – don't fall for it. Powerful people are trying to make you feel guilty for being human and you don't need to put up with that.

Conclusion

So, you've bought your flash new gear, you're bedecked from top to toe in Nike ticks or Adidas three stripes. You haven't eaten any sweets or cakes for a few days and you've been to several classes at the gym of your choice, or jogged every morning before work. You're starting to feel good, proud of yourself. You'll definitely keep this up. Life will be different from now on; you make vows that you won't lapse and allow old habits to creep up on you again.

You deserve a hearty pat on the back for getting this far. Try to keep enjoying your exercise programme; remember to take things as slowly as you need to and you will begin to relish your new found energy and self-confidence.

All you need to do now is keep going. Don't panic if you miss the odd session or if your routine is interrupted by a holiday or extra work pressures. Missing a week here and there doesn't mean you have to give up. Fitness is not a race with a finish line, it is a lifestyle which you will find to be constant and ongoing.

Get fit and you will definitely want to stay fit.

Good luck.

Other books in the Help! series:

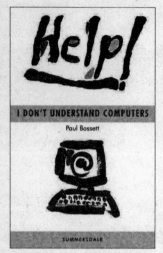

I DON'T UNDERSTAND COMPUTERS

Paul Bassett

SUMMERSDALE

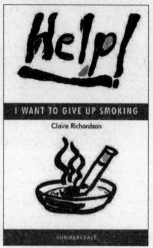

I WANT TO GIVE UP SMOKING

Claire Richardson

SUMMERSDALE

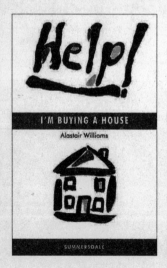

I'M BUYING A HOUSE

Alastair Williams

SUMMERSDALE

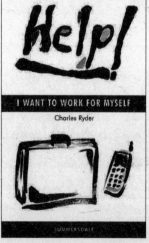

I WANT TO WORK FOR MYSELF

Charles Ryder

SUMMERSDALE